DIY Shampoo:
Top 30 Natural And Organic Shampoo Recipes

Table of content

Introduction

First and foremost I wish to thank you for downloading my book "DIY Household Hacks, Natural & Homemade Organic Shampoo Recipes for Healthy Hair." I hope you will enjoy using the collection of natural hair remedies that I have put together in this book for you to make use of.

Once you start to use natural products you are going to see a great healthy difference in the look and feel of your hair. It will no longer be bogged down and lifeless, or covered in unhealthy chemicals that are just stripping it's natural oils away leaving it dry and brittle.

The natural home remedies for hair products are going to get your hair looking wonderful and healthy once again. You can also share these recipes with friends and loved ones, who I am sure will be thankful to you when they too get great results from the homemade hair care recipes. Enjoy spreading the goodness amongst friends and loved ones with these great homemade shampoo recipes!

Chapter 1 – DIY Homemade Shampoo

Start being good to your hair, you can begin this by using some of the wonderful collection of homemade organic shampoo recipes in this book. Enjoy giving your hair some natural homemade special treatments. You are gonna love your natural look!

1. Cognac Shampoo. Cognac is known to do amazing things to hair and scalp. Enjoy this recipe especially when you see how great your hair looks!

Ingredients:

- one tablespoon of liquid castille soap

- one tablespoon of honey

- one shot glass of liquor

Directions:

Mix all the ingredients together and apply to hair. Leave on your hair for a few minutes then rinse.

2. Beer Shampoo. This homemade shampoo will bring shine and life to your hair.

Ingredients:

- half a cup of light beer

- two tablespoons of castille soap (liquid)

- one teaspoon of apple cider vinegar

Mix ingredients together put into old shampoo bottle and apply it as you would any other shampoo and rinse.

3. DIY Semi-homemade Coconut Milk Shampoo. This is a wonderful homemade shampoo recipe that allows you to make your own coconut milk shampoo. Your hair will look and smell great! I say semi-homemade because I use organic baby shampoo as part of the recipe. Even so this recipe is still much better than using store brand shampoos.

Ingredients:

- one quarter cup of coconut milk. Directions on how to make your own homemade coconut are below shampoo recipe.

- One third cup of organic baby shampoo

- one teaspoon of almond oil, or olive oil

- ten to twenty drops of lavender oil or tree tea oil

Homemade Coconut Milk:

Ingredients:

- one half cup of shredded coconut

- one cup of hot water

Directions:

Put the coconut and hot water in a blender and pulse about 20 or so times. Strain the milk into some kind of jar such as a mason jar, pushing down on the coconut to make sure you strain all the liquid out.

Put the coconut back into the blender with another cup of hot water repeat this process three times and you will be left with a jar of fresh homemade coconut milk.

Directions for Coconut Milk Shampoo:

Add one quarter cup of coconut milk and one third baby shampoo to bottle of your choice. Add one teaspoon of olive oil, and almond oil. Add ten to twenty drops of your favorite essential oil. Shake bottle now go and try it out!

4. DIY Shampoo for long hair. This homemade recipe is really great for long thick hair. Instead of using water this recipe uses tea. Did you know that Chamomile tea is a natural hair lightener? Try using green or chamomile tea. Enjoy your clean and shiny hair!

Ingredients:

- one gallon of brewed tea green or chamomile

- half cup baking soda

- three tablespoons of castille soap

- one tablespoon of xanthan gum

- essential oils about 20 drops of tea tree oil

Directions:

First brew the tea for your shampoo then let it steep for about ten minutes. Remove the teabags and add your baking soda. Let it completely cool down before you add your other ingredients. Add the rest of your ingredients then pour into a bottle to store in shower. Keep extra in a bottle under the sink.

This next homemade shampoo is good for helping with hair growth. For those looking for help in the area of growing their hair this might be the shampoo you are looking for!

5. DIY Vegan Homemade Shampoo. You can make your own vegan and paraben-free shampoo inexpensively. In this recipe castile soap, essential oil, and grape seed oil are combined. If you have dry hair add some aloe vera gel. If you have oily hair Tea tree oil or Lavender oil will help with that and will make your hair smell nice.

Ingredients:

- one cup of water

- one cup of liquid castile soap

- one tablespoons of grape seed oil

- one tablespoon aloe vera gel (optional)

- seven drops of essential oil (your choice)

Directions:

Mix all of your ingredients and keep in a bottle. It lathers really well you can also use it for shaving cream, so you are getting two uses out of this homemade product. If you have curly hair you may want to add some aloe vera gel for more moisture. If you have oily hair try using either lavender oil or tea tree oil with your shampoo.

6. Baking Soda Shampoo. This shampoo is great for getting rid of dandruff, and excess sebum.

Ingredients:

- two tablespoons of baking soda

- couple of cups of water

Directions:

Mix your baking soda into the water then apply this to your head and massage into it. Then rinse like you would any other shampoo. This will make your hair turn out nice and shiny.

7. Cucumber & Lemon Shampoo. The nourishing properties of cucumber and the cleansing properties of lemons is put together in this natural homemade shampoo. This will help to get rid of dry scalp.

Ingredients:

- one lemon peeled

- one cucumber peeled

Directions:

Put your peeled lemon and cucumber into a food processor or blender, blend until you have a smooth paste. Then apply as you would any other shampoo. Massage into your hair and leave on for a few minutes then rinse.

8. Cornstarch Dry Shampoo. Here is a great inexpensive dry shampoo with only one ingredient being cornstarch.

Directions:

Dab your roots with cornstarch if they look greasy then wait a bit then brush out and then you are done. Now how easy and simple was that!

9. Cornstarch Thickening Shampoo. Using the simple ingredients below will help to thicken the look of your hair.

Ingredients:

- one cup of water
- two tablespoon of baking soda
- one tablespoon of cornstarch

Directions:

Mix ingredients together to form a paste then apply as you would any other shampoo. This will help to add volume and thickness to your hair.

How about trying a natural shampoo that will do two in the one for you –giving you a shampoo and conditioner in one!

10. Shampoo for Dry Hair.   This natural shampoo will not only clean your hair but it will condition it at the same time.

Ingredients:

- one and a half cup of castile soap (liquid)

- two tablespoons of apple cider vinegar

- seven drops of Tea Tree oil

- half a cup of water

- few drops of lavender oil

Directions:

Mix all together then put into a spray bottle with a few drops of lavender essential oil. Apply to your hair by spraying onto your hair leave on for a while then rinse.

11. Homemade Body Shampoo.   This is a simple moisturizing shampoo made with three ingredients. This works well in cleaning your hair and body. Just combine the ingredients and put into a bottle with a nice shape or design to give it some added flare.

Ingredients:

- one cup of castile soap

- one quarter cup of coconut oil

- one tablespoon of honey

Directions:

Mix them gently in a bowl then pour into a nice bottle, and you are ready to enjoy some homemade shampoo that is suitable for your hair and body!

12. Natural Homemade Shampoo for Swimmers. No need to go to great expense on swimmer's shampoo you can make your own.

Ingredients:

- one liter of water

- two tablespoons of castille flakes

- one tablespoon of coconut oil

Directions:

Boil some water and pour in the flakes of castille, then stir mixture. Once it has cooled add your oil, then pour into a bottle and it is ready to use.

13. Anti-dandruff Shampoo. This shampoo is a great way to get rid of your dandruff naturally.

Ingredients:

- one quarter cup of distilled water

- one quarter cup of Liquid castille soap

- half a cup of grape seed oil or coconut oil

- one tablespoon of apple cider vinegar

- one tablespoon of minced garlic

Directions:

Combine all of your ingredients in a food processor, switch it to low and process until smooth. Now it is ready to use.

14. Lemon Shampoo a Shine Booster. This is a great shampoo if you want to get the shine back into your hair using a natural method.

Ingredients:

- distilled water one quarter cup

- one quarter cup of castille liquid soap

- two tablespoons of rosemary

- two tablespoons of almond oil

- half a teaspoon of lemon essential oil

Directions:

Make a rosemary infusion by boiling distilled water pouring it over dried rosemary and steeping it until cooled. Strain then use the liquid as a base in which you will add the rest of your ingredients. Bottle it and it is ready to use.

15. Aloe Vera & Lime Shampoo for Oily Hair. We all know that aloe vera is known for it's healing and soothing properties, this homemade shampoo is going to help to get rid of your oily hair.

Ingredients:

- half a cup of organic shampoo or half a cup of liquid castille soap

- two tablespoons of freshly squeezed lime juice

- one teaspoon of aloe vera gel

Directions:

Mix all the ingredients together put into a bottle and apply like you would any other shampoo.

16. Apple Cider Vinegar Shampoo. This great homemade shampoo will help to get rid of that dirty feeling kind of hair and replace it with some wonderful squeaky clean hair.

Ingredients:

- one egg

- two tablespoons of fresh squeezed lemon juice

- one teaspoon of apple cider vinegar

- a quarter cup of coconut oil

- six drops of tea tree essential oil

Directions:

Mix all of your ingredients in a blender, blend until smooth. Apply to hair massaging it in. Leave on for a few minutes then rinse with lukewarm water.

17. Avocado Shampoo. This homemade shampoo will help to neutralize your oily roots while nurturing your hair.

Ingredients:

- one ripe avocado pureed

- one tablespoon of baking soda

- one quarter cup of distilled water warm

Directions:

Blend all ingredients until you have a smooth paste then apply to your hair and leave on for 5-10 minutes then rinse off.

18. Egg Shampoo. This is a great simple recipe that will really help to moisturize your hair.

Ingredients:

- one large egg

- two tablespoons of baking soda

- two tablespoons of coconut oil

- two tablespoons of fresh lemon juice

Directions:

Beat the eggs before adding other ingredients then stir and mix. Apply to your scalp give gentle scrub then rinse.

19. Shikakai and Soap Nut Shampoo. The ingredients in this shampoo have anti-microbial and anti-inflammatory ingredients this is a shampoo that will make your hair feel and look great.

Ingredients:

- soap nuts 60 grams

- Shikakai powder one tablespoon

Directions:

Soak the soap beans in water and leave them overnight, then pour contents of your bowl into a blender. Add Shikakai powder blend, it is then ready to use.

Below is a collection of wonderful homemade remedies that will help you to get rid of that dreaded dandruff in a totally all natural way.

20. Salt It. Salt is something that most households have, but did you know that it makes a treatment for getting rid of dandruff? Because it is slightly abrasive it works as a great exfoliator, getting rid of dead skin cells and extra oils. It helps to clear the scalp off so that when you apply your shampoo it will be more effective. It is actually a very pleasant treatment that feels good, especially if you have itchy skin.

Ingredients:

* three tablespoons of Epsom salts or table salt

Directions:

Take the three tablespoons of salt and gently massage into your dry or slightly dampened scalp for 2-3 minutes. Shampoo immediately after salt treatment.

21. Aloe Vera Gel. Aloe vera gel is commonly known to help sooth burns, but you can also use it as a treatment for dandruff. The constituents of aloe vera gel inhibit the process of skin cell proliferation. Basically the stuff that makes up aloe vera gel helps to slow down the process of how fast your cells grow, dandruff is often caused because skin cells are growing and dying too rapidly, the aloe can help to restore normalcy.

Ingredients:

* one bottle of aloe vera gel

Directions:

Apply your aloe vera gel about 15 minutes before you wash your hair. Leave on your hair for 15 minutes, wash hair as normal.

22. Tea Tree Oil. Some oils can be the cause of dandruff, but other oils are helpful in keeping it under control. For centuries tea tree oil has been used medicinally. The Aboriginals of Australia used the tea tree plant leaves for treatment of burns, cuts, bites etc. There is fungicidal properties in the oil of the tea tree plant leaves. The tea tree oil is soothing to the skin especially when it is itchy or sore. You should remember that tea tree oil should not be ingested.

Ingredients:

- one tablespoon of tea tree oil

- one cup of warm water

- a squirt bottle

Directions:

Pour one tablespoon of tea tree oil into one cup of warm water in a squirt bottle. Shake the bottle well. After you have shampooed, spray your scalp all over with the mixture, massage, allow to absorb. Pat out the excess moisture but do not rinse out.

23. Lemons. Fresh lemon juice has acids in it that will help to break down fungus that causes dandruff. It doesn't cause any harm, as other man made products filled with chemicals and unnatural ingredients do.

Ingredients:

- two tablespoons and one teaspoon of lemon juice divided

- one and a half cups of water

Directions:

Massage two tablespoons of lemon juice into your scalp allow it to sit for a minute. In one cup of water mix in one teaspoon of lemon juice and rinse your hair with it. Repeat daily as needed. This will leave your hair with a nice lemony smell to it.

24. Healthy Eating. When you are eating healthy it effects every aspect of your well-being including your hair. We are learning more these days on how vital our diet really is to our overall health. So it should come to no surprise that it can have an impact on skin conditions such as dandruff. Below is a list of foods that can help you to get rid of the bothersome flakes of dandruff.

Lean Proteins. To try and minimize dandruff try adding more lean proteins in your diet. They help to build healthy skin and hair and keep it growing in healthy. Choose fish, and other non-meat proteins such as nuts, eggs, and beans.

Fish Oils. Using fish oil can make a difference in your overall skin's health. You can take fish oil supplements to help to reduce the severity of your dandruff.

Veggies. Our skin can be impacted by green leafy vegetables. Green veggies help to encourage healthy hair, skin, and nail growth. So try and add some dark leafy veggies to your diet.

25. Aspirin. Aspirin is probably one of the last things you would think of as a hair treatment, but the Salicylic Acid in Aspirin, is an active ingredient that is used in anti-dandruff shampoos. Salicylic Acid has anti-microbial and fungicidal properties, these will help to get rid of those awful flakes caused by fungus. Instead of buying Aspirin for a headache try it for a hair treatment. Crush a couple of aspirin in and put in some warm water. Then pour this over your hair and massage into scalp then rinse off after a few minutes.

26. Sun. There has been links to the exposure to sunlight and dandruff, but it is not exactly known why. There has been many documented cases that when people that were afflicted with dandruff spent more time in sun their dandruff lessened. Perhaps it is not dry weather in the winter that causes dandruff but the lack of sunlight. The sunlight may help to dry up excess oil on the scalp. It also just could be that the human body is enjoying being out in the natural sunlight, improving their overall health.

Directions:

Try and spend 10 to 15 minutes a day out in the sunlight. Don't spend too much time in the sun as the UV rays can be harmful to your hair, skin, and health. Like the old saying says "too much of anything isn't good." Moderation is the key in most things including how much time you spend out in direct sunlight.

27.   Listerine. When you think about Listerine you are picturing yourself gargling with it not using it as a hair treatment. But Listerine fights against fungus, and one of the most common causes of dandruff is fungus. Instead of throwing in your mouth try throwing it or spraying it over your hair.

Ingredients:

- Listerine (mouthwash)

- water

- spray bottle

Directions:

Mix one part Listerine with two parts of water. After you have shampooed your hair, spray the solution into your hair or scalp. Massage into your scalp and hair and roots, let sit for about 30 minutes then rinse your hair.

28. Neem Leaves. Neem leaves are known to be used as an Indian herb. They also make a great all-natural home remedy for dandruff. Neem leaves act as an anti-fungal, they will also relieve any itchiness you may have on your scalp. Some people find the smell of the leaves not very pleasant.

Ingredients:

- one cup of neem leaves

- six cups of hot water

Directions:

Put hot water with neem leaves in a bowl. Let the neem leaves soak in the water overnight. Strain the liquid and then apply this to your as a rinse. You may also try making a paste with the leaves, then apply to the scalp and let it sit for an hour or so then rinse off.

29. Fenugreek. Fenugreek is a plant that is used often as a spice in Indian cuisine, but it is also used for medicinal purposes as well. The Fenugreek seeds are rich in protein and are composed of amino acids. These help to encourage healthy hair growth and keep away the dreaded dandruff flakes. It has a high concentration of lecithin (a natural emollient) this can help to make your hair stronger, and feel silky and smooth.

Ingredients:

- two and a half tablespoons of Fenugreek seeds

- one large bowl of water

- something to grind seeds with such as a mortar and pastel

Directions:

Soak the seeds in one to two cups of water overnight. Grind them into paste the next morning. Apply the paste to your scalp. Leave on for about an hour, cover with shower cap, then rinse off with a mild shampoo or water.

30. Baking Soda. Baking soda is a great thing that serves many purposes, it is a good idea to keep some in your household. It is used in many natural home remedies and is cheap but effective in many home remedies. One of it's many uses is that it helps to remove dandruff. It will exfoliate the dead skin cells. It will also act as a fungicide and kill off fungus. It can also get rid of the loose flakes stuck in your hair.

Ingredients:

- one tablespoon of baking soda

- one cup of water

- few drops of rosemary oil or lavender oil

Directions:

For every cup of warm water add one tablespoon of baking soda.   Use old
shampoo bottle to apply the mixture.   Make sure to shake well before applying.
Instead of shampooing use this mixture, daily if you can.   You may find that your
hair feels dry at first, but your natural oils will restore themselves soon.   Your oils
will be much more balanced than when using commercial shampoos.

31. Vinegar. You may not like the idea of rinsing your hair with vinegar, but it
can be a real effective way to treat dandruff.   Dandruff is caused when skin cells
are maturing too quickly and dying too fast, it can cause great irritation. When
you use vinegar on your scalp it will get rid off dead skin, and it will not clog up
your pores and cause more dandruff.   It works like a fungicide.

Ingredients:

- half a cup of warm water

- half a cup of apple cider vinegar or white vinegar

Directions:

Mix warm water and vinegar together.   The amount may be varied depending on
how much hair you have.   Pour this mixture over your hair, rub it around your
scalp area for several minutes.   Rinse it out thoroughly with water.   Wait 8-12
hours before having a shower. Repeat the process one a week.

Here are some great natural hair treatments for those that are suffering from dry, frizzy, or dull hair. Using these homemade hair treatments you do not have to worry about them further damaging your hair, unlike store bought products that are filled with chemicals.

32. Amla Powder & Lime for Fuller Hair. If you would like your hair to look fuller try this homemade hair treatment.

Ingredients:

* one tablespoon of amla powder

* juice of lime

Directions:

Mix the amla powder with lime juice then apply to damp hair. Massage into hair and scalp leaving on for a few minutes. Rinse and shampoo as normal.

33. Soft Butter Hair Treatment for Dry, and Brittle hair. If you have dry and brittle hair why not try this homemade treatment using butter.

Ingredients:

* soft butter

Directions:

Massage butter into your dry hair and cover with a shower cap leaving on for 30 minutes. Shampoo and rinse out the butter.

34. Purple Kool-Aid. If you have brassiness in your blond hair you can do a rinse with grape-flavored Kool-Aid to get rid of it. I use this and it really works great I have never had my hair turn purple, but if you see any color just rinse again.

Ingredients:

- small package of grape Kool-Aid

- water

Directions:

Mix cool aid in a bit of water then add to your hair and leave in for a few minutes then shampoo.

35. Chamomile, Lemon Whitening Agent. This is a great rinse that will help to lighten your hair.

Ingredients:

- one jug of chamomile tea

- juice of one fresh lemon

Directions:

Mix tea in with some warm water and lemon juice then more over hair. Soak hair with mix and leave on for a few minutes then rinse.

36. Potato, Lemon, and Chamomile Brightening Mask. This mask will make your hair nice and shiny.

Ingredients:

- one small grated potato

- one tea bag of chamomile

- juice of one lemon

Directions:

Mix ingredients then apply to hair and blow dry for two or three minutes. Then, rinse and style your hair as usual. You will notice that your hair looks brighter and shinier.

37. Cocoa Powder Color Boost. If you have brown hair and need a color boost here is a great homemade recipe that will give you a deeper, richer brown color in your hair in an inexpensive but effective way.

Ingredients:

- one and a half cup of cocoa powder

- half a cup of plain yogurt

- one teaspoon of honey

- one tablespoon of apple-cider vinegar

Directions:

Mix ingredients together by whisking them into a paste. Shampoo your hair then squeeze out the water, and apply the paste. Keep the paste on for about three minutes. Rinse then style hair as usual.

38. Color Boost for Redheads. If you are a redhead here is a homemade color boost for your red locks.

Ingredients:

- two large carrots

- two tablespoons of honey

- three tablespoons of yogurt

- one cup of cranberries

Directions:

Take your carrots and finely chop them in a food processor or blender. Add the cranberries, and make a fine paste. Add the yogurt and honey and mix well. Shampoo then spread the mask throughout your hair, massage lightly. Keep the mask in for about two minutes then rinse and style hair as usual.

39. Pumpkin, Avocado, and Honey Hair Mask. This is a great way to use up the leftover canned pumpkin. Pumpkin offers many amazing benefits such as being rich in vitamins A and C, beta-carotene, zinc, and potassium.

Ingredients:

- one to two tablespoons of honey

- one cup of puree pumpkin

- half an avocado puree

Directions:

Mix Pureed avocado, pumpkin with honey to make hair mask. Wet hair then remove access water, then apply the mask to hair. Cover with saran wrap or shower cap, leaving on for 15 minutes, then rinse off. You can also apply this to your face for a great face mask too!

40. Tea Tree Oil, Banana, and Olive Oil Hair Treatment. Banana is a great natural hair treatment.

Ingredients:

- one banana

- one tablespoon of olive oil

- one teaspoon of tea tree oil

Directions:

Mix the banana and olive oil together mashing up banana until it is pureed add tea tree oil to the mix. Wet down hair and remove access water. Add banana mask and cover with saran wrap or shower cap for 30 minutes then rinse off.

41. Coconut Oil & Avocado Treatment for Dry Hair. If you have really dry hair try this homemade coconut oil and avocado treatment. If the coconut oil is solid put into microwave to make into liquid form.

Ingredients:

- coconut oil

- half a ripe avocado mash to a paste

Directions:

Mix coconut oil and avocado until you have a nice smooth paste. First rinse hair and take out access water. Then apply coconut oil and avocado mix to hair, cover with shower cap and leave on for about an hour.

42. Avocado & Peppermint Essential Oil Hair Treatment. This is a great hair treatment that will help to revitalize damaged hair.

Ingredients:

- half an avocado

- couple of drops of peppermint essential oil

Directions:

Mash up avocado into a paste add the essential oil and add paste onto damp hair. Leave on hair for about 15 minutes then rinse.

43. Purple Kool-Aid. If you have brassiness in your blond hair you can do a rinse with grape-flavored Kool-Aid to get rid of it. I use this and it really works great I have never had my hair turn purple, but if you see any color just rinse again.

Ingredients:

- small package of grape Kool-Aid

- water

Directions:

Mix cool aid in a bit of water then add to your hair and leave in for a few minutes then shampoo.

44. Olive Oil and Lavender Essential Oil for Dry Hair. Using olive oil is a good home remedy for dry hair it will put moisture back into your hair.

Ingredients:

- half a cup of warm olive oil

- couple of drops of lavender oil

Directions:

Warm half a cup of olive oil in the microwave do not allow it to boil. Add a couple of drops of lavender oil and mix or blend well. Rub into your hair and cover head with saran wrap or shower cap. Leave on for 45 minutes then shampoo and rinse.

45. Strawberries for Healthy Looking Hair. If you want a homemade hair treatment that is going to give you lovely looking hair then here it is.

Ingredients:

- seven to eight strawberries

- one tablespoon of mayonnaise

- couple drops of lavender oil

Directions:

Make a mash with the strawberries, mayonnaise, and lavender oil mixing up well. Apply this to damp hair then massage into hair. Cover with shower cap or saran wrap for 30 minutes then shampoo and rinse. You will be left with great looking luscious hair!

46. Sugar Water. If your hair is frizzy, mix some sugar and water and rub this into your dry hair.

Ingredients:

- one teaspoon of sugar

- one large cup of water

Directions:

Mix sugar into the water then pour some into palms then rub into your hair. This will give your hair a hold just like hairspray. This is basically homemade hair spray.

Conclusion

I hope that you will enjoy trying this wonderful collection of healthy 100% natural hair care products. You will see the difference in no time how great your hair will look when it isn't loaded with chemicals and other man made products that strip it's natural oils etc.

Not only will your hair look great but you will save a large amount of money making these healthier homemade hair remedies. You will have great looking hair that didn't cost you a small fortune to achieve!

Thanks again for downloading my book.